P.B.

# BEGINNING
## *of a forgotten*
# PROFESSION

## JOURNEY TO BE A VETERINARIAN

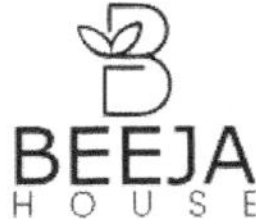



**ISBN** : 978-93-93635-60-0 (Paperback)

Any references to historical events, real people, or real places are used fictitiously. Names characters and places are product of the author's imagination.

Published by: Beeja House

First Printing Edition 2022
**Author Email**: pushproop@hotmail.com

# Contents

# Prologue

I am honoured to be given a chance to talk to you guys. I am in service of the animals. My call came in the late 80's when I enrolled in the profession as a student. Since then, a lot of water has flown under the bridge, a lot has happened. When I started the veterinarians were primarily expected to deal with large animals; mainly cows, buffaloes and horses. Things have changed and are a lot different today. Pets have become important family members

There are many reasons for this one important aspect is that Human society is ever changing and with that the needs of people have evolved. We are in times of nuclear families. Individuals and senior citizens need companionship. Pets seem to fill this void very well. There is an increasing emphasis on small animal medicine.

Unfortunately, in many countries like India Veterinarians are not taken seriously as professionals. I am not saying everybody is in this boat. Most people only assume doctors are only in human health and animal professionals are also doctors. I call this an overlooked profession. They are often underpaid and overworked and don't get the well deserved respect.

I have gone through this syndrome at home and in society. In this book and the series to follow. I am going to talk about how I enlisted and my journey. I am trying to make a pen picture of the journey spanning more than three decades. Reading this will give a lot more ideas of a forgotten profession. We forget how important this field is for the country and for the people.

In this book, I would like to share some interesting incidents via short stories. Things happened during my university days and beyond. I would like to inform the reader that even before enrolling as a veterinarian. I was always having a soft corner for animals and wanted to help them.
I would like to share an important anecdote, something major that happened as a kid, which shook my soul. I was helping my mother in her backyard poultry farm. I was young, inexperienced and very innocent. One day I saw a load of day-old chicks arrive. When I visited the pen I was excited and saw the young chicks run about in the brooder. They were day old, some may have the yolk still sticking on the feathers and I thought they looked dirty and my young mind came to a solution that they needed a bath.

I was not aware that the water would be that cold, the chicks had no way to control the body temperature and would actually freeze to death. Unbeknownst, to the consequence of my action, I proudly went up to my mother and told her what I did. Her reaction was naturally of shock, anger and appalling. Seeing this made me immediately realise what a blunder had occurred. Quickly returning to the barn I saw the floor littered with dead birds.

This caused a huge feeling of guilt and I started a deep introspection in my mind. I should do something to compensate for the error. These thoughts stayed with me till today and deeply affected me and also shaped my career. After all "thoughts are the seeds which define action".

ONE

# Introduction

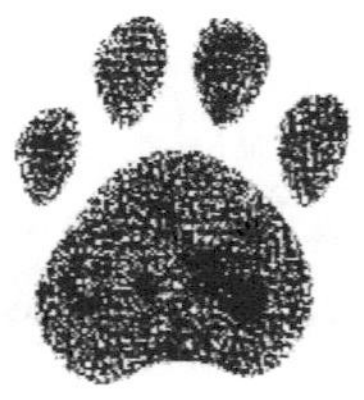

Life is a journey and whether we like it or not we will keep moving till the end. Time is the only important measure for this journey. We are on a one-way street, there is no rewind. As our train of life moves on, events unfold, new passengers come on board and some old depart. We also see people who just change the compartment and come back; others end their journey and are gone forever. We all keep moving on till our destination or station comes.

During this hectic journey what happens is called the incidents of life. Most of us fondly remember the interesting ones especially from our young days and the turbulent college times. They are truly memorable and can leave a deep impact on our mind and souls. Most college days are in youth and it is an impressionable age. These episodes can shape or reshape personalities.

The irony is that at that time when we are in the midst of the student days, we want it to end fast and we move on with so-called "actual life". When these days end and we step into a new chapter of life we are nostalgic about those times. Talking of college days makes a great dinner conversation for the rest of our lives.

These happenings could be diverse, vary from being pleasant, humorous, romantic, sour or even painful. The interpretation would be not what happened but how we reacted. The paradigm is very important, but then this is not constant and our feelings and interpretations could shift from time to time. What we find painful now could become funny later on in life or vice versa.

In this book, I present a very brief collection of stories about encounters or incidents at the inception of a new profession. We all know, it can be challenging to start something new. Especially, when we are young and the whole foundation of a new life is being laid. The profession is like an anchor around which our life revolves. There are mistakes which we make, triumphs, romances, good and bad people encountered. There are many new foreseeable and sometimes unforeseeable threats that could be faced.

My idea in writing this book is to relive and share the fun, adventures, excitement and even the turbulence of those times. Most of the stories are written for purely entertainment and also to give hope to the reader. It is not meant to ridicule, do character assessment or point any fingers at one. If some name or character seems familiar it is coincidental, they are not meant to be a caricature of any associate. My intentions are not to make anyone feel inferior or be picked at.

The journey is of a student in the late '80s to early '90s in Punjab. Was hard and could be turbulent. If we do the research, these years were extremely charged and were bloody. There were a lot of religious, social and political problems. The institute that was referred to here was at the centre of all this turmoil and thus, had an extremely unstable phase. Anything which occurred inside or outside the campus ended up creating a ripple effect which was loud and palpable here.

My sincere attempt is to put all this in a way that makes a good reading experience and many readers may relate to similar scenes in their lives. The place and times may be different but the essence may be similar. This essence is a very essential spice of life. We can understand this in a way that a story can be narrated which may create huge thunderous applause. The same story without the spice may be looked upon by others as downright boring. So, I have tried to add the ingredients to make the stories more readable.

I should own up, it took me more than 10 years to write this book. I had decided to write as early as 2010. Many times, I did start writing but lacked the discipline and the will to finish it. I easily got distracted, as they say life happens. In these years actually, a lot of things transpired. I moved, took a new job, started my business and also welcomed my second son. The old memorable incidents were so deeply etched in my heart and mind. This part of my memory cells containing the stories remained green and pregnant with episodes. They only wanted a chance to come out on the paper.

Before I close, I would like to thank Geetika Sehgal and Beeja education for providing me with the correct direction, boosting my spirit and wonderful guidance. It is thanks to then, I could muster the confidence to finish the adorable project. I am extremely proud and happy that this mission is accomplished. To some it may look like a small step but for me, it is a giant leap. As the Chinese saying goes, "The journey of a thousand miles begins with a single step. "

I hope I am able to entertain the reader and build a successful relationship. Here I would end by a famousI quote from a famous statesman, "This is not the end, not even the beginning of the end. But it is perhaps the end of the beginning. " I will certainly say the journey doesn't end here. I plan to write a series of more books about the journey so far. I am waiting for feedback to understand how I can get better.

# TWO

# Admission

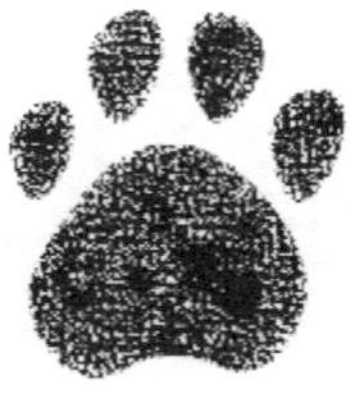

The admission to the Veterinary College was a natural consequence of my desire to serve and do something about the dead birds. It was certainly a new and uncharted path. I wanted to do something for animals. At that age you don't have experience and sometimes we make emotional decisions. Often we don't think or reflect too much. I wanted help out but never thought it would become a career.

When I enrolled I had already decided I wanted to join politics and was looking for a backup or set of skills in the field of veterinary just in case things didn't work out. In India, you had to choose a stream right after grade 10 and in those days the system was quite rigid. It was an annual system and it was not easy to shift from one stream to another. Theoretically you could but it was very cumbersome and time-consuming to take the deficiency courses.

While deciding it was not one simple factor, there were multiple things in my mind. I had the desire to help, there was a burden of having done badly in grade 10. This put me in the bad books of my family. I had to prove that I am a man and worthy of their trust. So, this became another factor to take up medicine. I did take up the stream but did not want to follow the same path as my family. I loved animals and the poultry incident was always weighing on my soul. it would be wrong if I don't admit it. I was also afraid of the intense competition and the time involved in human medicine.

I was juggling with different baggage, shaky and indecisive. I had a desire for great achievement but wanted to take the path of least resistance. I had heard some veterinarians do well and I justified it being a 4-year course and in the end, I'd be a doctor. I can serve the animals as I will have more knowledge. I will save the birds. This was a mid way point. I wanted to be an educated politician.

Our family had some ideas about the profession. We had a few family friends who were working or studying in the Veterinary College. So, this made the whole thing doable and inspired me even more. I had an inferiority complex and used to think, I am not at par academically, at least in our family. Mentally, I was under the impression that I can't achieve much academically. I had an average academic record, yet I acted as if I am street-smart. Moreover, I needed a degree though it was only temporary. That the chicken story was stuck to my soul. I was sure my final career was in politics.

One more thing which was always discussed in my home and I don't know what was the origin of this thought. My father and my grandfather both were physicians. They would indulge in bashing the standard of prevailing medical education. They had strong of the opinion that it is going down and incompetent graduates are coming to the market. They were critical of too many colleges and felt that there would be so much mushrooming of fresh graduates that they would not even get jobs. These talks were more out of their frustration but they created a negative impact on me.

This was the background and then one day, I was studying with my friend Suresh Kumar. I was scanning the newspaper and I saw an advertisement for admission to the local Veterinary College. I felt relieved and had a feeling of wow! It seems my problems are now over and my prayers have been heard. I now don't have to go through this gruelling competition. I will come out and help some birds and then somehow someone somewhere will pick me up to run for elections. Excited, I showed the newspaper and talked to Suresh. Shockingly he was less enthusiastic and looked kind of cold to this idea of applying to a vet school.

He was clear in his thoughts and said being a veterinarian doesn't excite him. He has some relatives but one he talked about. This vet is often smudged in cow dung. At the end he was clear this is not his cup of tea. He doesn't see the fulfilment of his dream job. His talk of a hand in cow bums actually made me think and for once discouraged me.

Now we have a problem, seeing the ad in the paper, I thought I had a solution. Now Suresh was throwing cold water on my dream. He is unable to understand my point. This is a cool professional degree and can crack it. The competition will be less. We will avoid the tough challenges and frustrations of failing to get into medical school. There is a reasonable career that too without much pain and struggle. At that time I was thinking a professional degree assures you a reasonable income.

I did not tell him so many things but my persistence and relationship convinced him to at least apply. I still remember I rode my bicycle about 7-8 km one way and went to the University to get two application forms. Then, I also came to know that my classmate *Kushpal P* is also applying for admission into the Veterinary College. This gave me moral support and made my case stronger. Now we had more company and someone I knew and respected..

So far it's good. Getting in there was a competition and we were supposed to take a pre veterinary exam Unfortunately, I made a mistake and I did not prepare well. I thought this exam would be a cakewalk. I was young and misjudged the situation. I forgot that competition is a competition. My thoughts were that I had spent years studying in grade 12. I knew everything and the level of the vet entrance exam should not be too hard. The second major error of judgement was in the exam, I did not attempt all the questions. I was just aiming to clear the test. This was a big blunder as there would be a merit list. In hindsight 20/20,

I wish I had not been complacent and worked hard at least in the entrance exam. My passage would be smoother and coming events will throw light on my fowly.

It was not that I did not have time to complete more questions. Every question left blank effectively means they are marked wrong and amount to a 0 mark. All this carelessness took a heavy toll and decreased my final score. When the results came, I was lucky to be amongst the top qualified candidates. But ultimately short of merit list. As per the accepted norms this exam was followed by the interview. The final results were a total of the written exam score, interview and suitability to the profession. The system was designed in a way that the interview favoured students who lived and took their previous education from rural areas.

During those days, the vet profession was designed primarily with an idea to suit the needs of farmers who had large animals. The state government was one of the major financiers and the priority was to boost the rural economy. Since dairy, wool, eggs and meat were seen as a source of secondary income for the farmers. They planned this education to be a technical and management support to the country folks.

Naturally, they preferred students who had experience dealing with animals. These graduates were more suitable and likely to go back and work in the villages. The interview was set upin way to be at a disadvantage to me. I had no rural background. My biggest hope was the written exam, which was worth 80% of the final score. The remaining 15% was for the rural backgrounds which as mentioned included education from a country school. The actual interview was only 5% which was kind of a grey area. The committee could favour a candidate if they found he/ she fulfils the needs.

I cleared my written exam and was invited to take my interview. On the interview day, we went to the venue which was the college. My dad's friend Dr M had been a great help so far in college. He always encouraged me emotionally and provided material to think about and prepare. The interview was held in the college's committee room. The room and the surrounding area were crowded. There were many staff members of the Dean's office, students and their relatives. As far as I remember, they asked me just one question in the interview: What is the use of horses? I don't remember my exact answer.

After all these steps, came the final merit list. I was shocked not to find my name among the selected candidates. I was 18th on the waiting list. I knew I could have done a lot better. It was very clear my lackadaisical attitude. Irresponsible preparation and the improper attempt had taken a toll and left me hanging. The chances of me making it from this position were looking very slim. Then, we know fortune favours the bold.

I was now adamant that I should get in. My self-respect was at stake. I felt I had something big to lose if I did not get in. I was feeling extremely embarrassed, upset and deeply hurt. As things unfolded something very favourable though unexpected happened. That year, there was a big strike by University and College Professors. So, the academic session got postponed and did not start on time. The classes usually start at the end of July and that year they did not start until October.

This delay caused many students with higher positions to drop out and the merit list moved on though at a snail's pace. Finally, it came to a point that I was the next candidate on the list. Here, we saw more drama happen. I was first on the waiting list and had a tie with one boy. To break the tie the authorities had no set formula. Suddenly they came up with a solution to use the marks of grade 12. This went against me and he was given the advantage. Contrarily, if he opted not to join, I would be in.

I could do nothing but wait for his decision. I prayed and wished that some miracle would happen. He would decline his position. The irony was that my parents prayed too. They wanted me to abandon, forget all this, give up my stubborn attitude and prepare again for next year's medical entrance. I had very narrowly missed getting into medical college. So they felt if I work hard I will make it. On my end, I was deeply offended as I had expected this to be a cakewalk I should get in. Here I am, struggling to get in and my friend *KP* is already in. I was happy for him but felt I do deserve to get in. I am struggling for every chance I have.

As this was happening, my father watched me run from pillar to post, he was further urged to act by my sympathetic mother. He was moved and finally came out to help me. He went to see the authorities. They were able to make contact with one gentleman *Mr R* who was in the admissions office. My parents did some groundwork. They dug up his background and approached him via close contact. Unfortunately, this fell flat, R was not in a helpful mood. so nothing much came out of this attempt. This gentleman R went beating about the bush and would neither make a decision nor would he commit. He was the guy who unilaterally changed the scenario by announcing a new formula for grade 12 marks. We advised him to use the marks of the entrance exam which was in my favour. In short, he was vague, abrupt and not clear about the possible next steps.

My father was now upset and that made him more persistent. He had a good network and knew some important people. So, he approached one more friend of his *SSG*. *Mr* SSG was a senior official in the state administration who happened to know *Mr R*'s boss. My dad and SSG went to see Mr Boss.

He looked at the file and *told R* if this tie boy is not joining, the authorities should act. They should adopt a more proactive approach and set a deadline. The other candidate should make his position clear and accordingly inform the authorities. He either deposits his fee and enrols by a certain date or he is out and the position is offered to the next person in the list.. After this talk, the administration did move but still at a slow pace. I believe it was more due to inefficiency than any collision.

After about a week or so, they did write to the boy and gave him a cut-off date. If he did not reply and did not come forward to deposit his fees, it will be assumed he is not interested. and the seat would be considered vacant. This boy appealed for an extension which after some delay got rejected. In the end, the tied boy did not join. But as a typical government office, they waited and waited. Why? Nobody knows.

Here my father made another determined push and this time he was able to break through and get the desired results. The list clearly moved on and I was finally given a green signal. Then, I quickly got the necessary formalities completed. My medical was done the same day as I got the orders. I still remember the doctor asking me to undress. Everything! Including the underpants! I was embarrassed though I was aware this would be coming. He asked me to cough. I believe he was looking for a hernia. The next day, I deposited the fee and I was officially in. I can still feel the euphoria. This was even better as it was a hard fought battle.

Here I should make a special mention, and thank my father's friend *Dr M* who helped me a lot in the whole process. Starting from preparation for the written exam helped me a lot even during the tricky admission negotiation. During my entrance test *Dr M* got a list of possible questions and also the answers for a specific part of the written exam called Suitability to Veterinary Profession. These questions were hard for me to prepare on my own. He based this on previous years' exams. These were questions like how many eggs a bird lay in one year, important breeds of cow, pig and such husbandry questions. I do admit this was certainly very helpful to me in the written exam. Later, Dr. B was helpful when we were running from pillar to post. He would give us moral support and valuable internal intelligence. He even accompanied my dad to meet some of the concerned officials.

This ended one chapter of getting in but started another chapter of staying in and successfully completing my course. My journey in the profession has been slippery like riding on a wagon of hay. As we have seen, getting in was tricky. Later, we will see it was hard staying in proved to be a big nightmare. I had underestimated the whole process. My academic performance was never my strength. This weakness showed up more prominently from now.

# THREE

# Academic Issues

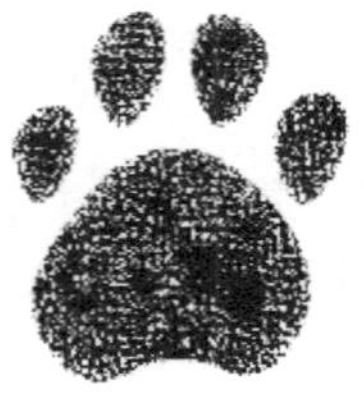

My initial year was very hard for me academically. I almost came to a point of being dropped from the course. The process of getting in was so painful and hard. It was shameful for me and very discouraging. I could never fully fill this void and the grades continued to harass me for the next few years. I still feel the pain and wish I could have focused on my studies and recorded a better performance.

I was a reasonably good student in grade 12 and as mentioned before had scored better and thus qualified ahead of many fellow students to get in. I was not that bad but my academic performance began to decline and came to a nadir. It brought me embarrassment and made me feel horribleI. My first exam was the statistics midterm test. I thought I was prepared well for the midterm and I was so confident that one day before the exam, I was out playing cricket. The next day, as I sat in the exam, I realised how wrong I was. My confidence was a false notion and things went topsy turvy and I struggled. I felt crestfallen like a cricket captain who lost by an innings.

 My other exams were also horrible. One after the other my players were being bowled out. I scored just enough to pass which effectively meant a poor D grade. The system was designed whereby if you get D you get 1 point, C- 2 points, B- 3 points and A– 4 points. So, passing and getting all Ds doesn't get you anywhere. One reason I thought was that I enrolled late and missed many initial classes. This pushed me out of the rhythm, secondly, I was never motivated to study. We had a lot of family disputes at home. This distracted my focus. If the lens doesn't burn.

To feel better and justify I was making all kinds of excuses. I did not like the environment or the end result in terms of employment after getting my degree. This degree suddenly felt inferior to my family standard. My thoughts were I will end up as a black sheep. It is hard to get up from being hit and get down. I discussed this feeling with my mother without mentioning the marks. She was frustrated with me and gave me the option of taking the entrance exam next year. This was also not something I was wanting to hear and was acceptable to me.

In short, I was scared, frustrated and confused. Unable to come to terms I became defencive and maintained the status quo. So I took the bitter pill and continued to do something which my heart was no longer accepting. I now think I went into survival mode. I tried to laugh off my pain and ended up being a class joker making everyone laugh. I would act confident and make witty comments and crack jokes but I was always afraid in my heart. I just could not and did not pay attention to academics. In short, my pain was so much I stopped caring, and I went into denial. I had a total mental block.

The mental block was something I have never experienced before and did not know how to come to terms. I would study, prepare and forget everything in the exam. It is possible my preparation was inadequate, did not revise the subject properly. This was a time of total lack of clarity. I also started preparing for medical entrance. This further robbed me of valuable time and energy. They would say you study one day before an exam. It never worked for me. It was a trimester system and exams come so fast. 1 st trimester, I got all D's except 2 C's. Next trimester I went further down, I got all D's. Now I was from the frying pan into the fire. I was in denial so I thought I could overcome this.

I tried to impress the teachers by asking questions and hoping to win their sympathy and respect to get good grades. I did go to talk to various teachers. I remember I went to the Professor of Genetics and he said you will get an A. Somehow, I failed to answer the questions properly and this PR exercise did not work. It was so painful and I kept failing over and over. Something I assumed would be easy had become a nightmare. It did affect my morale and to this day I can feel the pain and discomfort. It is funny how things work incidents pass but the feelings linger.

I was on scholastic probation and the academic rules stated that if I got below 1. 5 OGPA at the end of 1 st year. The university would consider me incapable of continuing and I would be dropped. To avoid this worst case scenario and boost my OGPA in the third trimester I had signed up for some repeat courses. These courses were considered easy and were a way the university would covertly help the students in trouble. Being an internal system the teacher would ask only what was covered. So in a repeat course they would purposely decrease the content to make scoring easy.

By now my name was on the watch list of the 18 students. These were the people who needed to grid up the lions or are gone. Overall I was discouraged feeling bad but still somehow had the brute confidence that this is a blip and I would make it. I saw some of my classmates' study for only one day and get an A grade.

In denial and to overcome the hurt I was doing other co-curricular activities. I attended the parasailing camp, NCC camp. These student activities normally are awesome to do but I was in serious trouble and these activities come at the cost of valuable time. In hindsight, I believe if I thought clearly I could cut my losses and spend the same time studying. This would certainly avoid my insanity of doing the same thing over and over and expecting different results.

In the end, I found myself in a situation where I was totally against the wall. In the last trimester, I had to get to overall 1. 5. I was considering all my options, covert and overt. During that day, my father's friend Mr SS G became the registrar and that was certainly a good omen. I used his help to get one grade lifted in FT. I got 66 but Mr Gill asked the HOD. A tough and very sincere person. He gave in and allowed me grace and I was lifted to a B grade. The situation was so bad It was my first B. I was jealous of my classmates who studied one night and got an A. My other classmates were doing so good getting solid A's and I was struggling. The question which kept reverberating- How were they superior and what did they do and why did they perform better?

One day as my final exams were coming to an end, one of the batch mates came over and said that I was on the academic watch list. As he was talking about this I was having a bad sinking feeling. my lips dried and I felt dizzy. My peace was totally shattered. I wanted to do something and something soon and wanted to be bailed out. As he left I got dressed and was getting ready to go and see the registrar. I felt he was the only guy who could now save me. He had the authority and was solidly behind me.

As I started getting dressed up my mother noticed something was wrong. I believe mothers are God's special ambassadors. They have a strong sixth sense and can hear and see things way before they actually happen. She asked me where I was going. I was broken and I definitely needed help and advice. I told her to see Mr SSG. She asked me why I was going to see him this late in the day. I confessed, "I am in a lot of academic trouble. " I explained the whole scenario.

I must confess a few days before this, I had even shamefully attempted suicide. I took sleeping pills as I had a very bad attempt at my final exam. Actually, the Stats exam and another exam were on the same day. I asked the class CR who normally sets the dates to change these clash dates but he did not do anything. He wanted to finish the exams and go home. He lied to me that the professor doesn't agree and won't shift the date. I had hoped I would manage to do well enough for a B, but it did not happen. I felt the end is here and started getting serious suicidal tendencies wanted to end my life.

My thoughts were that I had wasted nearly 2 years and this such a big mistake I have made. I should end my life and stop embarrassing my family. If they drop me I will have no option but to re-start BSc-2. What will my friends think, what will my parents and family think? This is such a shame. I would rather be dead than face this. I did not know where to hide and be in place so that i don't have to face the world.

 I went to the Pharmacy and bought sleeping pills. Those days they would give these drugs without prescription. The drug store guy asked me why I wanted it and I lied and said my family wants it. He gave me only 3 pills. If he had given me more, I would have probably taken all of them and not be here. I took all 3 pills and I remember I was so deep in sleep that I peed in the bed. This made my mother wonder, how come I did not wake up. I never told her the secret. After this, I did not attempt suicide again. I did some self-talk and decided to fight this.

Going back to the main story, mom wanted to help and the first person she talked to was my dad. Who had more resources at his disposal and he decided to step in. At that time all exams were not finished and I had one more exam to go. It was a very tough exam in Neuro-Physiology taught by a tough Professor *SSS*. So far I had assumed I would get an F in it. My father approached the Head of Department *Prof MSS* and also talked to the Prof SSS. I have discussed this in detail in another chapter. Prof MSS who now was aware of my situation secretly helped me and uplifted me grade to B. After this help, , I was clear but we did not come to know about this till many days later.

Another person who covertly helped me was Prof *HSP*. This guy was my anatomy teacher and also our NCC instructor. He happened to be the camp in charge for parasailing camp. He was impressed with my performance in the camp. In his anatomy exam, I could not answer any questions so I handed him a blank sheet of paper. This was a clear F but out of sympathy and humanitarian consideration, he awarded me a pass D grade. Which meant I passed and gave me 5 additional points. This help was not to my knowledge and I had expected an F.

So after my NM Physiology results I had cleared the magical 1. 5 barrier. This meant I would continue. I did finish my course. Some trimester I did really well but overall I was amongst the average students. Since the system was designed that every trimester counts I i never excelled or achieved my level of expectation.

# FOUR

# Physio

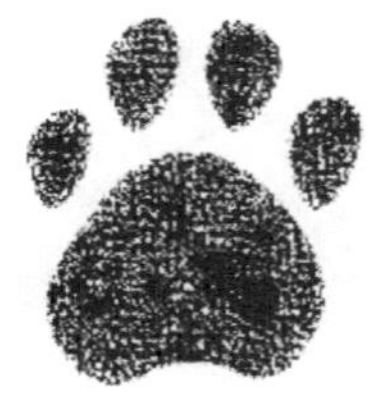

This 111 became a landmark event in my life as a whole and especially in my quest for my veterinary education. The first year, I was off to a bad start and was struggling with poor academic grades. This depreciation or decline in performance continued and at the end of the year or the third trimester, I faced a very big delima. If I did not qualify or get enough OGPA my academic education at this University would end. I was so close to being dropped. I was under a lot of pressure and upset and did not know what to do but certainly wanted a good ending like in Hindi movies, after climax everybody goes home happy.

In the midst of the challenge my mind was stuck and I was paralysed and could not focus and even simple things. Life had become a huge challenge. Till today I don't know why I passed through such a hard phase. Here I was figuring out a strategy on how to put brakes and to stem this rout. I was feeling like a poor farmer where every seed was dying.

I am not lazy but I have a weakness in that I tend to be easily distracted. In hindsight I think the only reason I had issues with my academic performance was that I was in double mind stepping in two boats should I continue or not continue in Vet School. I have discussed this before. I knew to be successful I had to plan well and as a student study hard. My paradigm was shifted to failure and nothing seemed to work.

Anyway, when I started the final trimester I was scared, still, something in me said I will make it. I consulted my classmates who were in a similar situation and I did take some repeat courses but mostly new ones. One thing which happened unexpectedly. My advisor who was to approve my course load. Causally looked at the sheet and asked me to drop a course as he felt the load was too much. I ended up dropping Animal Breeding. At that time we did not know what was going to happen. The whole class boycotted the final exam and was awarded A F. If I were there this would be a complete disaster.

Amongst the one new course, we had Physiology 111 or NM physiology. This was a really hard one. As things unfolded we got one of the toughest teachers who was also the hardest examiner. We called him miser as he would hate to give marks. When we started the trimester the Prof was new and it looked like I may have a smooth sailing. It gave me some respite and confidence. In between the teacher was replaced by a senior Prof who had a reputation of being a hard taskmaster. This proved to be a real nightmare. It looked certain I would fail.

At that time I was not sure if this would have a scary climax and end well or be a Greek tragedy. I was mindful of the development and tried hard to study and to get back on the line. I was studying the textbook and even saw the Professor a couple of times to get a better understanding and wrap my head around the subject. I remember asking him about something called "sham range". He explained it very well. Unfortunately, my luck did not change with all this and I did badly in the midterm. I was clearly not getting ahead. In the midterm I took the make-up exam and tried my best to prepare but as the results showed clearly in my face that my best was not enough.

In the midterm, I remember the day when I sat for the exam, and the paper was presented. I was suddenly blank and I could not understand what to write or even where to begin. When I looked at the questions it looked like I had heard the topic and read it somewhere. I could not remember it or write more than a few lines. One important and obvious reason was a lack of proper preparation and I had poor revision techniques. I felt like a person who meets his acquaintance after a long time or unexpectedly runs into a movie / TV star. They look so familiar but so different, you know that you know them but feel frustrated and can't recollect who they are and so can't talk to them.

In the midterm, what I did write was of very inferior quality. I am ashamed to say that out of frustration I did cheat. I don't justify my action but so did others. I saw one of my classmates was openly coping from the notes he brought. The young teacher tried to stop him and he would not listen. Seeing all this, I was encouraged and started coping. I ran out of grace and I was caught by a senior Professor. They wanted me to stop and took no other action. I pointed out to the other guy they did not throw any of us out, only took our material away. After that, I was more confused and shaken and could not write even a single line.

You can understand my mind set and my morale level after doing all this. I went to my friend *HU's* house. I told him what happened and he was excited and said, you guys will score 100% marks. I did not muster enough courage to say, we will do good and get 100%. I came at best 50% which was barely passing. In the end, I didn't even get passing marks. The time bomb was ticking and my position was becoming soft. I had to get the OGPA to survive but it was looking gloomy by the hour.

The examination system was designed in such a way that no single exam would decide the grade. For every course we had several exams: the first hourly was usually worth 10%, the midterm 25-30% practical 25-30% and the end term remaining completing upto 100%. In the case of 111, there was no first hourly and we started directly with the mid term. After poor performance in the midterm, I had fewer options left. I had to make up for the loss in the practical and end-term.

The train of time is moving so all dates like platforms arrive. We reached our practical date. I I wanted to do a good and create an impression in the oral part of the practical. This would straighten up a few things. The senior Prof was taking the oral exam. He asked me three questions. I was not blank and answered all three. I remember one question he asked me specifically about what neuron synapse is?I tried to explain but I did not come out with the exact definition he was looking for.

In the end, I thought I did a decent job. It was better than my attempts in the previous trimester. In those courses they would give you passing marks even if you just gave a smile. We used to call this toothpaste advertisement. My thoughts did not matter, it was his thoughts which were decisive. There was obviously a big mismatch between the expectation and my performance. He gave me a zero in the oral which again was a setback and was taking me further away from the requirement.

To cut the long story short to pass or get a lowly D I needed at least 70% in the end term. That would just get me a 1 point and if i did not get D i was getting a 0 point. This teacher was clearly a tough task master. The miser was giving marks not dollars from his pocket. As the end term came closer it was looking like a monster and I was peeing in my pants. The problem with end terms was all the exams would have back to back. I could not cope with it. I again took a medical excuse and applied for make-up.

Since I took the make-up I would get little extra time to prepare. I heard the marks awarded to all the classmates are generally low. The situation was so deplorable that even the topper had scored just 75%. So, I had a truly uphill battle just to pass. Failing was not an option here. Now, I was losing my confidence even more and in this situation truly affecting my morale. I was wondering how on earth I could get 70% to just pass. When others who usually did so well were struggling. At this stage, I came to know after totalling my other courses that D alone won't be enough. C grade was mandatory or I am out.

To get a C grade, I needed to score more than 90%. Wow! This was certainly becoming even harder. Like a tailender is on strike and he suddenly realises he needs 30 not 18 runs out 6 deliveries and facing the toughest bowler. I was thinking what chance do I have when the brilliant boys and the cream failed to come close. The students who were just cracking the exams and always getting more than 90%. If I get dropped by what my family will feel and say, my friends will laugh at me. How will I cover this up? My future will be dark and I have wasted so much time. I remember I was now a 19 year old broken man and was under a lot of emotional stress.

My mother got wind that something was wrong. My mother is a fighter and I know her personality. I knew she would not keep quiet. She took my elder brother and they met Prof who in turn verified the details and apprised them of the exact situation. Things which even I did not know about the exact marks required. I did not know what to do next. One thing was quite clear: my effort alone will not be enough. Past records are the best indicator of future performance. It was amply clear I will not be able to do it alone and will need a lot of help.

Now, my father was given a briefing and he also stepped in the ring.. He is a great organiser especially with academics and loves a career oriented agenda. Releasing the gravity of my case he took charge of the whole situation, he then asked my elder brother to also chip in. The latter was in med school and had a good understanding of these complex concepts. Fortunately the NM physiology is quite similar in animals and humans. The team was formed and we all agreed to give the best shot possible. This now ended up becoming a family affair. Ultimately a history was about to be made here. Failure was not an option we had to make it a Hindi movie.

I remember, we studied the notes which was the whole course several times. We studied the material repeatedly and line by line but I don't know why we missed one vital part, a big diagram which caused me some difficulty. I will get to this later.

I would compliment my father for the initiative. I always had faith in him and knew he was a good teacher. His techniques were simple and doable. He would take up the subject and divide it into parts. Then make you go over it again and again. This helps you revise it several times as you study and your confidence goes up. We all know Repetition is an important part of memorising any subject.

This technique makes the hard frozen topics thaw and they flow like water. I remember as we went on my morale was getting high. At times, I would go back and ask the Professor questions and clarify my doubts. He was sympathetic, responsive and helpful. To help us out he even gave us an old question paper which proved quite valuable. I think I was lucky I had a good focused support team. I also got about 10 extra days to prepare. As the exam came closer, our efforts increased.

On the day of the exam, I was at ease. I reached the centre on time. I was in the washroom and I had a urinal chat with one of my cohorts. He was nosy and asked me how many marks I needed to survive. I was not expecting this and did not tell him the correct number. As I feared, he would make a comment on it and could be harsh. His cynical words would break my heart. I lowered the requirement and he still said this is pretty hard for you, can you do it? I told him I was working hard. His next words were hard work alone may not be enough. I ignored his words but could not forget them to this day. So obviously it was hurting.

In the exam, I was well prepared and had a great start. Everything seemed to go in a clock-like precision. I was going to crack this. I got stuck with the part we took lightly. There was one chart/ diagram which we had missed almost everything else I knew. Somehow, my team had likely taken this diagram lightly. I did review this a couple of times but not really like a solid preparation. I kept going and finally, at the end of the exam I knew, I had made it. In the end, I scored more than 95% during those days, a very tall order. If I had prepared the chart, I would have certainly scored 99%. Which would be a new record for this Professor.

The consequences of the exam were good and pretty far fetched, not only did I survive. It raised my self esteem. Opened doors for better grades in times to come. Next trimester, I did way better and scored good marks. I could not have visualised that I could do so well. This also included an A grade.

So this 111 was a watershed course, a life-changing event, I remember it as a landmark event in my career. Starting as the worst nightmare, a definite F as a family we focused and worked on it and ultimately hit a jackpot.

FIVE

# Birthday Parties

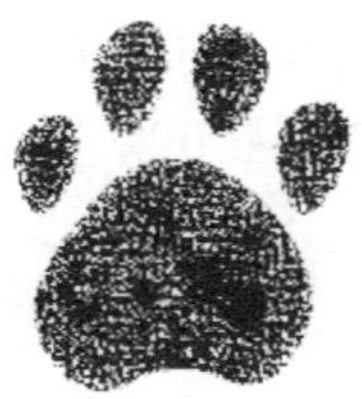

We used to celebrate the birthdays of our friends and would host a party in a well known local restaurant. It was a lot of fun. We had good food and a great chance to meet up. In those days we did not have cell phones and did not take too many pictures. This party deal started as a small group of 3 and grew to 9-10 class fellows.

In our vet school, we were basically 2 kinds of students: locals and hostellers. Having a similar background of being a day scholar we formed a kind of informal party group. Our youth needed some activity and soon started organising birthday parties. I don't know exactly how it started but it was really exciting and something we looked forward to. It was awesome as long as it lasted.

Maybe, I was the pioneer and organised a party for my birthday at the best local restaurant. My friend *Harish U* hosted a party at his house. I don't remember if this happened before or after my restaurant party. It doesn't really matter who was the harbinger. During those days, this eatery was considered one of the best in the city. Our city was an industrial hub and had some good rich people. So, we had some fancy dining places.

I have very fond memories of my first party, attended by 4 boys. Those in attendance included Yours truly, *Baljinder G, Rod C* and *HU*. I decided to throw this party taking a leaf from my brother who was known to host and attend parties. At the first party we had a wonderful relaxing time with some good food. My friends did what all party guys would do to get presents. They did this very covertly. I did not expect or want any gifts. I have a clear memory of two 2 neatly packed books: one was the Guinness book of world records and the second was a novel. Those days, there was no internet and printed books were more common. No offence, I don't remember the title of the novel, I don't recollect. It is possible that I did not even finish the novel.

It was funny how they secretly kept these presents hidden till the end. After the delicious meals, the duo *RC* and *BG* excused themselves to go to the washroom. I and *HU* were waiting in the restaurant. Suddenly, I noticed them walking towards the parking lot. Naively, I pointed to *HU* where these boys were going?. He was part of the conspiracy and lied. His words were I don't know, I did not see them, maybe it was someone else. Even after having seen them and heard an unpalatable excuse, I still did not suspect anything. I thought maybe something came up and they will be back soon. A few minutes later, they are back with something in their hands which was obviously the presents. I was totally flabbergasted and refused to accept the present. They really insisted and I was left with little or no option.

I was thinking this to be a one-off event. Did not expect this to become a trend. Soon, other friends joined in and all of us began to organise similar parties. It was certainly more exciting now as we had to get together at least once a month. The group grew in size. Friends began to invite other friends, mainly from the same class. When we started the number was 4 then it became 9 or 10. Since we were all from the same grade we were familiar and knew each other well. The host had the freedom to invite anyone, even an outsider. But the core remained the same; it was those 9 or 10 boys. As the group became bigger we had more fun but it had the usual effect of politics.

The event was always to celebrate the birthday. So, we would try to coincide and host it as close to the actual date. However, It was not always possible. Sometimes, we had exams or we were busy with something. We would organise at the earliest mutually convenient date. As far as the agenda was concerned it was similar. We had a dinner party at the same restaurant. I don't have any recollection of a birthday cake ever being cut. During those days, we did not have the culture of the hotel giving candles or even the claps.

As far as the food was concerned, most of us enjoyed non veg, meat or chicken. One of us was a pure vegetarian. When his veggie dish came, it vanished quickly and non-veg dishes were still hanging around. Veg dishes were mainly mixed vegetables or something of paneer ( cottage cheese). In those days, non-vegetarian food was mainly chicken or mutton. After the sumptuous meal, we would still go to a local food hub to have a dessert, mainly ice cream. We found the ice cream prices in the restaurant expensive. As a student, the money is always tight. We did not work and we were financed by our banker; parents.

Along with the party, we designed the system of presents. Most of us did not want to spend too much money but *HU* had high tastes. The presents were certainly cute and of good utility. This went on for 3 years and I must have received at least 3 presents. I have memories of jackets, one was a blue denim one and one was a green cloth jacket. We would pool the money and then one of us would go out to do the shopping for the whole group. By default or design, mostly it was *HU* who took the lead. This present deal did affect our budget and make the whole thing more expensive.

As mentioned we had distinct personalities and there were differences and politics. We did the party but we were not really one homogenous group. The common uniting factor was *HU*, who had a unique leadership quality and a rare ability to bond all the boys together. He really was good at making new friends. I had never known this quality till I met him, and experienced this first hand. I am sure if he was not in the group, we could ever have had these dinners. Not all days scholars were part of the group. I don't remember if *KP* ever joined us or was invited. He ran on a different frequency and we could never gel well.

There was an incident which happened during our celebration. I can't forget it. During those days the state was going through political law and order challenges. The state was in the grip of a wave of militancy. Adjacent to the restaurant was the office of the city police chief and the main interrogation centre. One day as we sat having our dinner there was a loud sound of gunfire. Thisshooting was obviously very close. Hearing this set the management into motion. As a safety measure, the restaurant shut off the lights and asked everyone to lie on the floor. There were at least 5-6 rounds fired and then there was silence. We remained on the floor for a long period. As long as the management did not feel it was safe. It was close to 15-20 mins but it seemed like forever.

We were all very young and even this firing was taken more like a joke, and we laughed at it. At that time, we never realised someone could have been shot or even have died in the crossfire. We did not know what happened, who was the victim or the aggressor. It was very apparent someone attacked the police station or the police fired at some suspicious element. Even the media did not cover this. There was no news about this episode in any of the newspapers.

The mystery was cleared decades later. I was watching a YouTube channel and realised that the firing was done by two militants who were targeting the son of the police chief. This boy had come out to smoke and was spotted by the passing militants. These militants had a grudge against the father but took it out on the accessible soft target, the chief's son.

Our parties did not last forever. All good things do come to an end. Our bashes could not go on forever. The group had strong undercurrents and it had to split and these parties were to finally end. The last party happened in my absence. *HU* always had an idea and would want the party to be organised on the actual date or close to the birthday. *HU* also had a soft corner for one *Venkat* and wanted to make sure he came. Sometimes, he even went the extra mile to keep his childhood friend and neighbour happy. Like giving him a ride and even setting a date as per his convenience. Ensuring V was not dropped or forgotten.

During this party, I was away and coincidentally before leaving I called *HU*, informing him that I am out of the station and I will be back in 2 days. Unbeknown to me they organised the party in my absence. On my arrival, I came to know that they had celebrated the B'Day. I was aghast and was deeply hurt. I felt left out and as if I had no relevance. This was too much to take.

I did not keep quiet and raised my objection to the whole process. The host *RC* feigned ignorance since he was kept in the dark about my phone call and also pressured to host it the same day. Innocently, he gave in and he was also not aware, I was away. I know he was correct and was telling the truth. He had no reason to lie. Only *HU* was aware that I was unavailable. He did not tell anyone and lied to the whole group. He told them I have been called and that nobody answered the phone at my house. During those days cell phones did not exist, so the only phone we had was the landline. There was no way to prove if someone called or nobody answered.

This was the last party nobody ever talked about restarting the process. There were multiple reasons including the fact that we were ending our education and priorities were changing. The sense of unity never matured to a level that boys would want this to go on. The cost of presents was certainly a factor as I heard some members gossip about why we need to spend on expensive presents. Frankly, I liked receiving the cute presents. Overall It was fun till it lasted. A cherished memory, something which I will never forget.

SIX

# College Fights

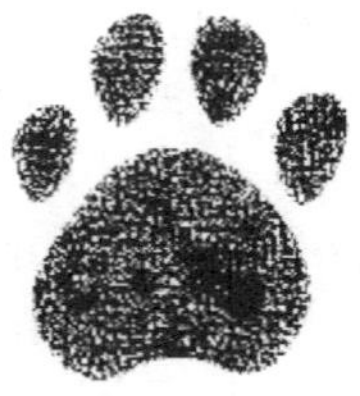

When I joined the University, I knew it was notorious for federations, fights and student disputes. The place stands witness to many major student turmoils, including armed fights and has been infamous and associated with gun violence and student death. I was guilty of having enrolled in my college with prior knowledge of all these facts. Coincidentally, during my student days, the militant political drama was at its peak. The university because of its student and staff demographics became the hotbed for all of these scary and unwanted activities.

The district administration and local police felt this was one of the key points of a potential serious backlash. The philosophy was if they can manage to keep this campus incident-free, half the city's law and order problem is solved. We witnessed many student strikes and frequent boycotts of exams and classes. This was facilitated by the education system which was internal.. All the exams were conducted by the same set of teachers who were also the instructors. So, the timings of exams were flexible and based on mutual consent. I had seen exams happen, even weeks after the trimester/ semester officially ended.

In many university unions the students were divided into groups who often fight for domination. During my days, the radical right-leaning Sikh federation was the dominating body. So, many would dress up and feign to be the members of the federation. Students irrespective of ideology would ape the appearance with long uncut beards. I know of students who would suit their personal interest and jump from ideology to ideology.

A few years before I enrolled the communists or left-leaning student organisations held sway. During those days, the institute had tragically seen a few murders of students and even some senior officials. All this was a reflection of and influenced by the atmosphere and events in the state. I was so innocent. I did not understand why there are these factions in the academic institute and what good they serve to improve the quality of education and research.

I have seen and it was an open secret of these student leaders misusing their position. They would threaten the teachers to get grades. They would leak question papers and steal answer sheets. Years later, I came to know how they ran the nexus.. They had influence and would smuggle out these exam questions. One of my classmates told me a story about how he used to go to the hostel one night before and there he would crack these tests. Then they would either memorise or make chits.

This movement was bloody, and almost all the state was affected. Some innocent people inside and outside the campus were jailed or even killed by the police or vice versa. Then it always happens manipulative and shrewd boys misused the charged atmosphere to their advantage.

Not all disputes were based on ideology, some were common law among student groups. The first incident of a violent fight that I witnessed was shocking. I saw 2 motorcycles with 3 boys each holding naked swords storming into the college. They soon attacked a couple of students. I am not sure how many were attacked. I saw two college guys gushing blood after being attacked. One was attacked on the head. He was bleeding and was rushed to the nearest emergency hospital. This was very scary and made me uncomfortable. I could recognize one of the offenders. He was my junior. Though to date, I have never asked him what happened or why did you attack?

I would generally avoid confrontation and physical fights. I had an ideology based on humanity but am more non violent. I would twist and turn around my words in a way that it would look funny and no one was offended. I was basically not timid or afraid of all this and I never understood the logic of violence. A couple of times attempts were made to drag me into a confrontation but I would successfully get out of it. Not bow down to pressure but negotiate my way out. One advantage which I had was that I was a day scholar and most disputes happened in the hostel. During the day, mostly you have your classes or are involved in educational pursuits.

I should say once a twice was dragged in. Every time- my no confrontation policy didn't work. In short, you are not lucky every time. One incident happened in the college which I can't forget and I was trapped without me wanting to be trapped. I got into a tricky situation where I was attacked and had to stand and face it. This happened because a junior student got so mad with me that he wanted to physically settle it with me. He wanted to teach me a lesson for having insulted him. Which I never did?

I used to participate a lot in debates and declamations. I was considered the best in college, at least for all of the English language events. Few students even attempted to participate in these literary activities. Mostly I was the only participant who represented my college. There was one more boy who was interested, he was *Jag G*. We were not the best of buddies, we were kind of friends but not the bosom buddies. He would often participate and many times we did share the stage. He might have been intimidated by me or was holding a secret grudge. Something which I can neither confirm nor deny.

A very minor incident precipitated into a physical fight. One time, we had a competition in a neighbouring city and I had an invitation to go. I was given the option to choose my partner. I was a pretty cool guy, so I did not care who would come with me. Actually, I would be ok with *Jag G* but his name never came into my mind. I was thinking of taking a girl student who had shown interest. I did not take her as I felt it was inappropriate, or even scandalous as this was an overnight sojourn. She had openly expressed interest to come with me but I deliberately did not take her. We lived in a conservative society and it would be misunderstood and could be interpreted as flirting.

I took another relatively unknown boy who was recommended by my friend RR. Like I said It was not important who would come, I needed a warm body. Overall, I was myself not very enthusiastic to go. It was like I was being forced to show up. I reached the venue with this boy as my teammate. I was already feeling uncomfortable and left the event before I took the stage. I made an excuse for a family emergency and took the next train back home.

I came back and started my usual student activity. *JG* must have gathered the information and was not happy, he may have even thought I purposely ignored him. His thoughts were wrong as I did not ignore him. I don't know why he got these ideas. He confronted me and asked me why I did not take him with me. I felt rather taken aback and almost felt threatened. I was not very keen to answer him because his approach was very condescending. In my mind, this was not a case of personal enmity. It was my choice and there was nothing wrong with it. Moreover, in the past, he had never expressed an interest. He was not even a close friend. I don't remember what I said to him or if I was in any way threatening or insulting. I must have said something that did hurt his ego or he was feigning a situation to create a fight.

As I came out of the college building, I saw 3 boys sitting on my parked scooter. One of them was *Jag G*. I knew all of them as they were my juniors. It was clear from their body language that there was trouble. I was not afraid and did not run away. I came directly to my parked vehicle. As I came to start my vehicle the trio pounced upon me. It was an uneven fight 1 against 3. There was not much of a hitting, it was more symbolic. One of the boys was a close friend's friend and he actually diffused the situation by saying ok... ok... This was enough to diffuse the situation and they all moved away.

After that, I was thinking there could be another attack. So I was doing my defence preparation. Make it public, become a victim and create as much noise as I could. I told my close friends they promised to join me if the situation did become physical. We were the seniors and they were the juniors. The hierarchy was certainly strong. I know I must have talked to 15-20 students. I am not sure if this did something, created a favourable tide or acted as a buffer. The matters calmed down and there was never a mention of this again. There never was another attack. I don't think it was on the agenda. *Jag G* and I ended up becoming friends.

I still don't understand why students get involved in these fights. I know sometimes tempers are raised, ego's get flared but there is always a simpler and an honourable way out of it.

# SEVEN

# DG

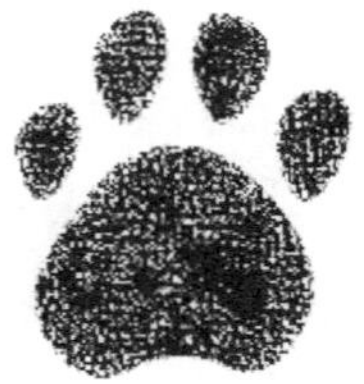

We know life is unpredictable. It has many twists and turns. We must have all experienced an event that can lead to totally unexpected results. I am going to tell a story along these lines. Which is to me is very fascinating and romantic

This happened to me in the city of *Banglor H* with a beautiful girl, Depti *G*. The story started with our team's participation in a national level youth festival. This invitation to this event was new and totally unexpected. Along with the dance and music events they were hosting literary events. I had a good reputation in these activities like declamation debate and quizzes. A few weeks before the team was announced I had won a prize in English debate at a university level youth festival. So I was naturally a star and was expected to represent the college.

On my part, I was reluctant to be part of the team as I had been to a lot of festivals. I had my fair share of travel. I was also under pressure from my family to stop going out frequently. Anyway, Dr *PN D* convinced me to sign up and go. I was actually called by the Dean to his office. He saw my past credentials and advised me to represent the college. As per his opinion I was the most suitable candidate.

I did go to this national tournament organised in *Bgl*. The first event was a debate. I was to speak on a topic and was given 24 hours to prepare. As I finished my speech I was sitting with a group of students enjoying the cultural show. I met a couple of girls. One of them was *DG*. She was an Asian ( Chinese ) girl. We hit almost instantly. We started our coquettish conversation. It was the first meeting and she did what many girls would do, encourage, smile and indicate their interest but not open up or show they are reserved

I was thoroughly enjoying myself and wanted the time to freeze and this time to last forever. I should be in this awesome frame and all this should not stop. The company and the whole atmosphere were really pleasing. Alas! This did not last and soon it was time to go. I was feeling unhappy about our parting ways. I was still feeling satisfied with myself as this was the first attempt. I was mentally looking forward to how to take the relationship further.

I was not nervous and the whole conversation went smoothly. After this encounter there was a different kind of current in my heart and soul. Mostly, I don't have a mindset for starting or building affairs. For such things I am kind of a very aloof guy. I was never into these things. This seemed to be different. Everything flowed naturally like a stream of water. After the first encounter my mind was focused on how this encounter should be taken to the next level.

When I came back I became her penfriend. I started to correspond with her via letters. We had no email, no social media, snail mail was the only available platform. Surprisingly, she responded very warmly and we exchanged mail for nearly one year. About one year later I went back to see her in *Bgl*. She was cute and very pleasant to talk. She received me warmly and we spent a good time together. We went around the city and took her out. She was very sweet and seemed to be quite understanding.

I must have gone back and forth 3 times. The ironic part was that the travel was not easy and often involved a complicated system of seat reservations. It was a 2-day journey. The most popular and affordable means of travel were railways. During those days, the system was not fully computerised so the reservations were to be done from the station of departure. This means the day you reached *Bgl* you had to make an attempt to book your return journey. This did not seem to bother me at all. I was focused like an archer on a target.

My frequent visits and our correspondence definitely blossomed the relationship. We became closer and it got better. As the romance blossomed I came to know more about her. She was actually seeing another guy from Ethiopia and was sleeping with him. I was not upset because we never had any commitment. But, I did tell her that she had to decide if she wanted to continuewith me she had to break off the relationship with that guy. She instantly agreed but later seemed to be reluctant to take action. It is possible she did not want to break his heart or was not sure if our relationship was stable and will it be worth it. She finally broke the relationship but continued to meet his contacts.

She finally graduated and decided to go back to her home country *N.* I somehow wanted her to stay in the back. I had the feeling of insecurity that if she goes away, she won't come back. Her environment would change and she will be influenced by her family and friends. This will definitely affect her priorities and it is possible she may break up or just fade away. That will be the swan's last song and will be curtains. These thoughts made me very uncomfortable and I was determined not to let this happen and to keep this relationship alive.

So, I figured out her hot button and advised her to try for a PG at my *University*. It worked. She got excited and applied, and she was invited for the interview. At that point, I thought she would be selected and this would be a simple process. I did not know that tables would turn and it would become so hard. The stumbling block and the main issue was she was a foreign national and the rules were different. I knew about her citizenship but at that time, my impression was once she got into the PG course all the necessary formalities and permissions would just follow. Unfortunately, that was not what happened. The university was located in a disturbed area and at that time foreign students were not allowed. A lot of government clearances were required and it ended up being quite complicated.

The department and the academic branch of the university accepted her. The Head of the Department was happy to take her as a student in the master's program. The registrar office was to oversee the whole process. It was to follow the ministry regulations and would not clear her name. They wanted a letter or clearance from Delhi which was a serious issue and very cumbersome to obtain.

At that time, I had no contacts in Delhi. Which was turning out to be a major bottleneck. I was adamant and did not give up so easily. I approached the ministry and tried to get an assent. I remember, I went to my friend's father who had some contacts. He was helpful and even deputed a staffer to drive me around and see what can be achieved. I went with this guy in his car to see the concerned officials. We met a couple of people who mattered. The feedback I received looked promising. I was confident that I would take time but I would be able to get the necessary permission. This would take time and would involve a number of departments but was certainly not curtains and there was hope.

As I was working on this file, I did not realise there was another story developing behind me in my blind spot. She was getting frustrated and was under pressure from her family. As per the initial understanding, if selected she was supposed to come by a certain date to pay her university fees. The issue here was her candidature had not been cleared and she would not be eligible to be enrolled. I told her not to come and wait for all the i's to be dotted and t's crossed. The whole situation was a little confusing and she was unable to fathom the depth of the challenge and being under pressure, she was losing her cool. So, without discussing anything, she started her trip.

 She was already halfway on the journey and she called me from the border. I was stunned by the development. When she called, my first reaction was to ask her to go back. She decided against this and still proceeded to come down. When she arrived, she was angry with me. I was accused of being rude to her on the phone. I was not expecting her to come down like this. I was trying everything in my capacity to help.

Her trip failed which was expected and she went back empty-handed without any achievement. The authorities would not budge and had their hands tied behind their backs. All this affected our relationship. I got a big jolt but did not end it here. The relationship was now clearly looking gloomy and sick but was not dead. I was having a double mind and clearly, she was getting cold feet. I did not give up and travelled to *Kath* to see her at least 3 times. I could clearly feel she is getting more and more aloof. It was apparent her focus had changed.

She soon joined the police and at that stage, the writing was clearly on the wall. It is hard to say but it is possible she may have even started dating someone else. There was one guy who was hanging around her.

Whatever was the case I had the feeling of having lost her. There were a number of instances where she totally ignored me or she would even purposely try to belittle me. On my visit to Kath, she would ignore me. I would keep waiting in the room with no phone call or message. Her tone and attitude were changing and I could sense that in her behaviour and body language. I don't deny the fact that on occasions she was warm, we went to see the Dussehra which was a very big show. The king and Queen were there.

Finally, I decided to let her go and stop pursuing her. I have a simple philosophy: just let go if things are meant to be they will come back. If they don't the things were never meant for you in the first place. Here it never came back and finally the passionate affair just came to an end. She stopped responding and moved away a few months later. I came to know through a mutual friend that she was going to get married.

Hearing this I was a little upset, a little not wholly crazy. For a brief moment I thought I was misled and cheated. What should I do, go back to see her or call her or at least write to her. I did not do anything as my soul advised me pushing her is like whipping a dead horse, it will never get up. Going to see her is out of the question as she will only make me a jack ass and she could get me into a lot of trouble in a foreign country.

 Even if I do talk to her, she will either ignore not going to answer or out of frustration say something which will hurt me more. If I write she will certainly throw the letter in the dustbin. If she did not care to keep up the correspondence what was the level of any feelings in the heart. This is life not a romantic novel.

This was the end of my first romance. It is life on planet earth. Things happen and hearts break but life goes on.

EIGHT

# Green Guy

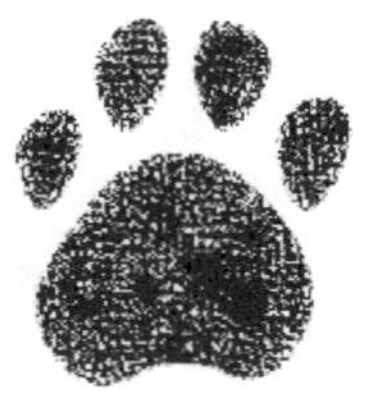

The story can't be complete without mentioning PCF 345. The adventures and stories of PCF 345 can be viewed in different shades. It was cool, funny, stupid and even tragic. I am trying to adopt a wholesome approach. Making it easy to read, not too heavy stuff

It was like a family tradition that we got a scooter or motorised two-wheeler after 2nd year in a professional college. My elder brothers got their scooters in Medical college. My story took a little different turn. I was supposed to continue on a bicycle in the first year. Things had a different turn. My new green coloured cycle was stolen from my home. My family was not willing to invest in another cycle as this would be temporary and end up with an unnecessary vehicle in the house

This theft became a blessing and I was approved for a scooter right away. Initially, I got a used scooter but then I was soon given a brand new light green coloured scooter PCF 345. As a family, we had purchased 3 vehicles in a short period of time. Two scooters and one motorcycle. My father's friend was in an important position in the district, so we got the VIP licence plates or vehicle numbers.

This vehicle or also called guy served me well and was abused by a number of my friends. This guy worked with me through thick and thin. In good times, bad times and also kind of stable times. I used to liberally lend it to my friends and acquaintances. So, not only I but many of my buddies had memories associated with this two-wheeler. There are many interesting and funny anecdotes associated with it. If it were not for this guy, a lot of things would have happened in a different way.

When I started using this vehicle for college many students and staff did not have the luxury of owning or driving a scooter. Many would just use bicycles to work. In those days, scooters were just getting popular. Some students and their fathers used to share scooters/ motorcycles. Their family would own it and they would borrow and use the vehicle on a need basis.

My guy was a light green coloured Bajaj Chetak and it had 4 gears. I had the pillion wheel removed as it was the fashion in those days. The indicator lights came in late models. After a few years of abuse, the groves on the gear shaft did not remain crips. A change in gear would make a jarring noise. Friends would joke and say my guy had numerous gears 35-36. Over time the scooter suffered from multiple other problems. I will discuss later how the shockers gave way. I got the breaks fixed many times. Many of these problems were associated with rough handling.

It lost its rear shock absorbers and driving became hazardous. I don't know how I noticed the problem, what triggered the red flag, and who or why I was advised to visit this specific mechanic.

After having looked at the various issues he came to the conclusion the rear shocker needed to be fixed. I had no idea what the shocker absorbers were and what role these shockers played. When he said, "this part has to be fixed or the guy could suffer more damage. " I was stunned and in total disbelief. The estimate seemed to be high and I had the impression that I would just add gas and never need any repair. I don't know how many times I even got the oil change service done. I was always trying to be cheap and cut corners

I am embarrassed to say, "I was so frugal, I didn't even buy the foot mats. " I was cheap and wanted to buy the minimum equipment and skeletal spending. One day, a class fellow jokingly pointed out that the bottom looked naked. I should get the guy appropriate clothes. I was not expecting this comment so I did not feel offended and I just laughed it out. I had no plans to get anything suggested. This statement still reverberates in my mind after decades so it must have created an impact.

One moist winter morning, my scooter skidded. The reason is that the tiers, especially the rear, had lost their groove and become totally bald. I knew the problem was coming as the rear wheel bears more maximum weight so it was worst affected. I did get the tire rotation done. Later, this rotation also will not fix the problem. The options were either to get new tires or get them re-treated. I did not have the budget to get new tires. My mother would mostly finance all these expenses. I remember that during those days she would always be tight. So, I did not have the guts to ask her for the money.

This neglect caused the bald tier to lose grip on the road. On a wet road, I skied and fell on the road. Luckily, there were no major injuries to man or machine. The bystanders felt I was badly hurt and came to help me. I was given a ride home. I felt comfortable, with no broken bones or pain anywhere. It only showed how careless I had become and the machines required adequate and timely maintenance.

This guy served me well and often I made him do more than recommended. I had bad habits and would often get late for my class. I would then ride this guy really fast. During those days the traffic was way light so I could get away with it. There was one particular turn on the campus that was tricky and scary. This was quite acute and the risk of slipping was high. Though I never had an accident here. When I turned at high speed I extended my knee and would dream I was in a motorcycle race. If you watch them on a turn they always extend the knee to get an adequate balance. I did that and thank god I escaped every time. Slipping on that spot could have resulted in a serious injury. Even now, I think I was lucky to avoid this disaster. The centripetal force at the turn could have easily spun me out. This would probably make me fly off and hit the road could have even hurt my head.

Accidents did happen with this guy either due to my carelessness or my friends' mistakes. One day, I asked my friend *Rajto* to take the driver's seat and I was in the pavilion. I don't know if he volunteered for this or if I opted to do this. Whatever the reason, he was driving. Right from the start, he seemed to be a bit nervous and shaky. I think he lacked experience which was affecting his confidence. Soon, the worst happened, he lost control and we skied. I hit the road and injured my wrist and there were bruises on my body, especially the arms. Fortunately, this crash happened close to the hospital. I quickly went to get the bandage done. The paramedic put my arm in a sling. This cost me miss my games.

One day, this guy *Rocky* borrowed my guy and ended in a major accident. My guy had weak brakes that did not work as expected and he hit a motor car, he survived major injuries but was badly damaged by the vehicle. He survived and thankfully no human got hurt. *Rocky* proved to be a good-hearted guy and he owned it up and he offered to pay to get it fixed. He first gave it to a random mechanic. I was angry with him for the accident and the consequent condition. Then I thought in the given circumstance what more could I do. I even contemplated telling him to forget to pay for the damages. Then I changed my mind and decided that he is at fault and should pay. I decided to take my vehicle to a known body shop. It was expensive to get the repair. *Rocky* stuck to his promise and he did pay for the denting painting. After this, I kept using my guy for several years. Never realised I still have an ongoing issue. Later, when I sold the guy, I realised all the broken parts were not completely fixed.

Years later, I had decided to retire/sell my guy. There was a tailor who worked close to my place of work. He offered to buy it for me. I was so desperate that against my mother's wishes, who was the actual owner, I made a deal. My negotiation skills were poor and it was one of my weaknesses. I agreed to his quoted price and that too was in multiple instalments. Overall it proved to be a bad deal for me. He got the guy checked and found the damage, this was the first time it was to my knowledge. So, he got a point and unilaterally paid less. I could have pushed him for this was something new but I did not. All these negotiations were never approved by my mom. I feel guilty. I let my mother down.

Riding and using this guy taught me many valuable lessons. One thing which I understood was that the gas price always rises. When I started my university study I could buy a litre of gas for less than Rs. 10. 00. This would last me for 3 trips.. Gradually, the price kept going up and in about 6 years, it had tripled. In the scooter, they added petrol and a little engine oil. If you use pure petrol, it would mess up the engine and it would seize.

Talking of issues regarding gas, during these years we had the first Gulf war. This was the time when President George Bush senior attacked Iraq. The consequences of the war were far-reaching and we saw the gas pumps become totally dry. There would be a few stations that had a supply of gas. Soon there were long queues at these pumps. Many times, I used the white lab coat trick. The attendants often assumed anyone wearing a white coat is a doctor. This would get you a priority and could jump the queue. Then one day this white coat game stopped working. I was at the pump and the owner was not present. He had a better self-image and refused to honour my white coat. I was upset as I was always given a priority at this pump. Then, I saw a friend of mine getting served ahead of the queue. I knew him very well and having failed with a white coat now wanted to use his name, but I was blocked again. The owner was not giving in; he seemed to be becoming arrogant and rude. The issue became not only did he decline service he used insulting words. This I felt was not fair, polite and actually very rude

During this crisis, we started seeing 2 lines based on gender. Separate for men and women. Of course, the lady's line was short. I often had to wait for long in the Q to get my turn. Frustrated with this one day, I asked my mother to help me out and stand in the short line for me. She declined because she was into her social activities and was prominently known. She found it embarrassing to stand like this with a scooter. Next, I turned to my grandmother who was more than 70 years old but she agreed to help out. While she was in the line, I heard some bystanders notice an old lady with a scooter. They obviously knew this was a hoax. They began to comment and I heard these whisper about this. I did not stay silent, I owned it up as it is from my team. In my heart, I did feel embarrassed that I am making an old lady stand like this. I never did this again. I felt thankful to my granny but felt bad at myself for taking advantage of her age.

There were other advantages I had with my guy. It was used to try to form bonds with my classmates. I had a feeling that I needed to keep my friends happy to avoid harassment. Many times in the past I had been ragged, especially at my school especially when I was young. This experience stayed in my heart, so I was afraid I could again face a similar situation. Our mind has the ability to create scary scenes. To avoid it, I used my vehicle as a tool to create a good rapport and avoid any unfriendly ragging situation. In my mind, I was thinking if I appease them they would not make fun of me. This was not totally correct.

There were other students who were in a similar position of ownership but they were more conservative. I am not sure how many bonds I made but I definitely paid the price for this attitude of propitiation. I don't know who I used my vehicle for. I heard some stories of this being used to courier girlfriends and even call girls. There were other stories of how I had to wait for long hours in the hostel or college as my scooter was being used by someone else. During those days, we did not have cell phones or tracking devices. So, if someone has your vehicle you have no idea where he/ she is. Then the so-called creditor was running his errand while the owner waited.

A few university mates used this guy like a guinea pig to get experience and confidence in riding. One of them, RR, was a short guy who did not like sitting behind me as he felt I blocked his view. So, he asked me to sit behind him like a pillion while he acted as the chauffeur. I was so naive and a people pleaser that I agreed to this ridiculous demand. He basically used me and my guy to gain experience. I know I should have stopped it but at that time I just lacked balls and went with the flow.

This green guy PCF 345 was a very interesting story. I can write on and on and have a full book on this vehicle. I still remember many of the experiences I had. Both inside and outside the campus. I don't know where this guy is. Maybe scrapped or standing in some garage somewhere.

NINE

# Speaker's Form

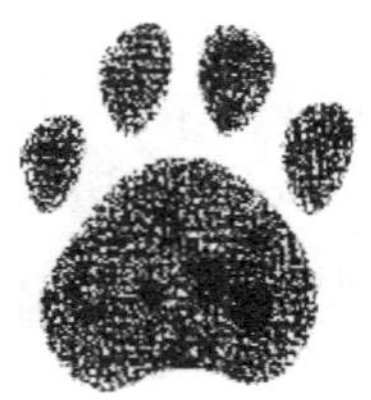

Life is a roller coaster always in motion. We experience many twists and turns and times come when we can suddenly feel on top you have encountered a new talent. Something which was there in our hearts but due to distractions or lack of confidence was never able to focus. It remained in oblivion and was never palpable. A single incident can change the scenario and we are able to prove to ourselves and show the world that it existed in our bosom.

This was something that I experienced in my university days, later making me feel like a star. It started more or less accidentally. One day I saw a poster about an elocution competition being held the same day. It was part of an intra university youth festival. I leapt in even though I was not prepared. I boldly stepped forward and participated and got the 3rd prize. It was for the first time in my life I stood on stage to speak and was recognized for it. This did great things to my confidence and morale. This event opened more doors for me and felt people listened and this pleased my soul. I decided not to miss any chance to be on stage. I participated in as many local competitions as possible.

My commitment was amply supported by the president of the speaker's form. *Dr. Prem D* Initially I was only participating and getting a very few prizes. Still, it pleased me that the thrill of holding the mike and speaking in front of an audience was outstanding. Mostly, my work was appreciated though this appreciation fell short of the judges. I actually started thinking, I am very talented. I want to be a politician and this is my training school. I mostly spoke in English as I had more control over the language. Though you had the option of speaking in Punjabi and Hindi. I was stuck with speaking in English. This acceptance by the audience made my mind fly high with ambition and confidence. I wanted to try more competitions.

One of the biggest events came in my life when our University team participated in something new called the Interuniversity Model Parliament. Initially, we were asked to participate in the event and we were not provided clear cut directions. We had a vague idea as to what it would be like. So, we started preparing using a rough guidebook. It was the only tool provided by the Bureau of Parliamentary Studies and Training. The training was under the guidance of one Prof Joe. We knew this was something to do with the procedures in the Parliament. The Bureau was reaching out to the Universities who are considered to be the seed of the future leaders. It was an attempt to sink the ideal democratic values in the heart and mind of the students

We did some initial training and prepared with what he thought would look like some informal discussions. We, focused on the current issues and things which were being talked of or likely be an issue. Like the education policy, agriculture problems. We were forbidden to discuss controversial issues or use it as a form to condemn or endorse the government stand. We did understand the structure of the government, opposition and knew there was a President, Vice President.

The book did give some insight and various procedures in the parliament, role of the speaker, parliamentary decorum. How the bill was introduced and debated and then passed. It was advised that we present, debate and pass at least one bill. We were lucky we had a student who was an experienced debater and a strong personality *Jug*. That girl had guts and was a born leader. She could handle situations and make people dance at her fingers. When we started she was one of the only leaders everyone looked upto. But as the process went on many more leaders were in the pipeline.

To make matters easy and more efficient, we decided there should be two groups: the opposition and the government. So, the floor was opened to the participants to volunteer for whichever group they wanted to join. The opposition was always more glamorous, romantic and it is easy to shine when you criticise the policy.. In opposition, you have more chances to say anything with force. It gets more claps and media public attention. I however chose to be in the government. I feel I will do better in the treasury benches. My thoughts were that I am good enough and should look for a constructive role.

After a few days of rehearsal it happened as always, the event was indefinitely postponed. So, we are back to square one. Now nobody was clear if this would happen in the near future or even happen at all. So, we all stopped our mick drill and dispersed. As we would see, some of the students in the camp lost interest. One of the participating colleges did not come back at all.

I was not thinking on those terms. I saw it as a chance to work with one of the top talents. Here, we had the best students from our university, later we would have had a chance to work with national level student speakers. *Jug D* and a few other colleagues were like hot stars. There was no doubt this was very good form and provided some awesome learning opportunities. My confidence went up and my talent to speak on a larger platform was sharpened. I also honed some important leadership skills, formed many new friends, some of even lasting me for a lifetime. This also gave me a chance to understand people and how to deal with human resources.

The first challenge we all faced was how to select a good team. The tournament rules specified we needed a team of 30 participants. There would be certain roles earmarked like the speaker who would be conducting all the activities thus in the main spotlight, president who gave the opening speech in English, the vice president who spoke the translation in Hindi, head of the government was Prime Minister and his cabinet, leader of the opposition, staffers like parliamentary secretary, guards and few other supporting members.

As a college our thoughts were that we wanted a fair representation. There was a need to avoid domination by the most populous college. This could in tum mean that all those who were not students of this college would be sidelined. So, it was proposed that we have equal participants from all the constituent colleges. This will give it more credibility and reflect inclusiveness. To my surprise, this proposal was unanimously accepted without much of a debate. This rule means that we will also have 6 seats per participating college.

After a few days of rehearsal it happened as always, the event was indefinitely postponed. The ugly scary head of delay and uncertainty was looming on the horizon. So, we are back to square one. Now nobody was clear if this would happen in the near future or even happen at all. So, we all stopped our mick drill and dispersed. As we would see, some of the students in the camp lost interest. One of the participating colleges did not come back at all.

I had not totally given up, I had hope that this event would happen. It was not clear when? I wanted this to be staged but the question was how soon, will the dates clash with the exams. As luck would have it a few months later *JD* showed up totally unexpectedly in my class. I was very happy to hear when she said the program is on and we are meeting again. I was excited and we started practising seriously. One of the participant colleges showed no interest in this rejuvenated agenda. They ignored our repeated invitations. This walk out changed the whole dynamic. We were now allowed to have the seats vacated and the number per 7 per college went up to 7.

The question was where to get the 7 students who will be willing to participate. The debate and declamations are by default considered dry subjects. I wanted to recruit so I actively started asking friends and classmates. I got 4 of them to agree they were from my class. One of the boys was proactive and got 2 more candidates from the junior class so we were meeting the past quota of 6. The new 7th place which was recently created and was still up for grabs. So, I got my friend *Raj S* to sign in and with this the team was now complete. Most of our team members were not effective public speakers and were silent backbenchers. The 7 boys including me never formed a very cohesive team and were often fissured.

While we were finalising our team other colleges were putting their list forward. Later, we had the students from management studies. These candidates were smarter and I would admit did lift our overall standard. They were more aware about what was happening and vexed for debates and discussions. It was not true that others were dumb or living in dark well.

Getting the numbers as required we started preparing to the best of our ability and understanding. Every working day after classes we would meet for a couple of hours and brainstorm. We would discuss potential questions worthy of discussion in the parliament. There were no YouTube videos available, the live television coverage of proceedings was still not approved. So we had to tax our imaginations, we were guided by a few available books and some material sent to us, especially about the decorum and procedures. Soon, within a few weeks we felt we were ready to go.

As we were getting ready we were hit by another administrative hurdle. The university authorities began to block the permissions. One day before, it was Sat and the final signatures were withheld. We should have a female teacher as young girls were in the team. Luckily we had some experienced players like *Sam S.* He had contacts and skills on how to deal with these issues. He was resourceful and self motivated he quickly took charge. He began to use his talent and tapped his contacts. He went to the administrative block and tried to iron out the existing objections. Seeing him I was also motivated. I could not sit back and be a silent spectator, I jumped in this struggle.

Regarding the issues concerning student safety and the girl participants, I had expected Joe to show his magic but he miserably failed. Now it was up to us students to ask one lady teacher to sign up. We worked hard and finally got one of the female teachers to agree. She had interest since her daughter was also in the team and *SS* had a good relationship with her. *SS* had past exposure and was part of many drama teams; he was a known person and definitely knew how to pull the strings in the university. Today If I look back I can say if it were not for him and his selfless hard work the whole episode would be over. No team would go as the necessary clearance to participate would not be granted. This would be 'The End'.

After the lady teacher was arranged we needed a vehicle, possibly a university bus. We did not have time to book train tickets and even if we did it would not give us the flexibility and privacy. I clearly remember just 30 mins before the university closed on a Saturday afternoon. We got the OSD to sign the dotted line to depart and also take the univ bus. This OSD was not a cooperative person. He had an attitude and also was very unsure of what to do. Several times he threatened that he would not sign and he raised a series of objections. Finally, we talked him into getting his precious autographs.. So here we had overcome two main objections of the bus, and the female teacher

There was more drama unfolding on the morning of our departure. As I came with my suitcases packed and ready to go we realised some of the team members had developed cold feet. One of the MBA guys said something very cheap which was not suited to his profile, it actually shocked me. His talk made me understand he had no idea about the developments. He said since the lady teacher is not decided and the girls can't go so he is not excited to go. It was not time to argue we just updated him.

Undeterred, with the current development and committed to the cause, yours truly and SS are now set about to meet this unexpected and sudden tsunami. Getting the team participants together. We asked the lady teacher, Mrs K, to accompany us and she agreed. *SS* and *JD* had a strong influence on her. We then went about getting the rest of the team to meet at the spot. We had no cell phones and even the land lines were primitive so we had to go from hostel to hostel and also some homes had to be tapped. Then we went to arrange for a cooperative and available driver and make sure we got the allotted bus.

After all this effort another unforeseen twist was in store, we got the bus but no money was allocated for the fuel. The question is what do we do now - cancel the trip? We were more committed and had worked hard to reach here so we all decided to find a way out. We voted to pool in the money for fuel and all the sundry expenses. At the time of this decision, we were all made to understand that since we are the official team representing the university our expenses will be reimbursed. We will surely get the money back. If this was not the understanding I am sure many of us would have backed off and we would have The End.

Later, due to audit objections, this did not happen. Years later I found out that the audit objection was a routine process and they had just wanted more clarification before the bills were cleared. This did not happen and the students who presented the bills did not care. By the time I got briefed and started moving on this information it was already too late to do anything.

Anyway, all said and done we reached the destination and lucky we had some boarding and lodging arrangements. It was one big hall or were there two halls I don't remember? There were beds in these halls and we had to take our beddings. For food there was a mess which served breakfast, lunch and dinner. This was all in a hostel booked by the university authorities.

During the entire trip, especially more in the beginning, I was not in a good mood and was edgy and would constantly flair up. I felt I was being sidelined and not given my due importance. I had a good hold over public speaking and was talented but was being totally overlooked in the main decision making process.

The MBA students were dominating the whole show. During those days, MBA had a lot of value and these guys acted as if they were divine and knew everything. There was one person *Mr Garry S* who was an experienced person and he was nominated for the position of the PM. *Jag D* though not from this group had very good natural leadership qualities and she was the speaker. Another MBA guy was the leader of the opposition. I was to be the minister of Agriculture.

In spite of all the preparation we did, there were doubts about what the final presentation should be like. Struggling and confused, the team made one wise choice, we decided to approach the organisers. They listened to the problems presented by the team representatives. They advised us to sit in the audience and watch the performance of other teams. This role of the spectator came as a big blessing. There were many valuable insights gained.

Like we did not know about the role of President and Vice President. This address and the translation of the opening speech was acquired from here.. We also understood how the opening parade was to be enacted. We did not know anything about the role of the Secretary-General. There were other issues with the bill presentation and the discussion which we learnt.

All said and done we did our best and with God's grace, and surprisingly we won the first prize. This was clearly beyond our expectations. We had always felt like an underdog, we were like the cricket team of 1983. When we started we had no idea who our competitors would be and this was our maiden attempt. This could be our first and last attempt.

This victory was certainly achieved thanks to tea effort. There was a valuable contribution to the maturity and professionalism shown by people like *Jag D* and *Mr. Gray S*. I am sure without these wise people, we would have been at a big loss. Our attempt would be average at best. This zonal victory was significant to our morale and boosted the team's confidence.

After this, we were to represent our university in the national finals. This was very good news and to be upto standard we had to prepare harder. Our victory though a welcome thing did create a lot of ripples. We were poorly rated now, the novice team suddenly looking like successful veterans. In the finals we decided to retain the same team. Our thoughts now were to keep at bay, hostile people who did not believe us, ridiculed or ditched us at the last moment.

A few months later we participated in the finals. This took place in the same venue and has similar arrangements of boarding and lodging. There was less red tape and bureaucratic hurdles from our university. In the national finals, we were placed 3rd with a bronze medal. That was still an achievement, something good to talk about.

In both the zonal and finals I retained my position as a cabinet minister of Agriculture. I observed these MBA guys were smart, they dressed up sharply and were more lively on the floor. I, however, did not even take my tuxedo suit and tie. I made other errors like I did not practise my answers. While speaking I was more extempore. I was good but still showed weakness of good rehearsal. The tournament had some individual prizes. I never was good enough to win any individual prize.

This was not the end of the game. This was now staged as an annual event. I participated in the next year's zonal and finals. The following year, the zonal round happened a little far. Now we had the services of Dr. *PN D*. He was a very good organiser and was able to use his influence to get a lady teacher, a good bus and gas money. In short, as a good manager he did all the expected groundwork. We also got better treatment from the university.

This year we travelled longer and we had more fun on our journey. I was not able to deprat with the team as my brother was getting married. To join the team I had to take a train journey. We were not sure where we would be the loding. I was following the main team soI had asked my friend to call me and let me know where we are staying. I provided him with all the necessary information about my train.

He acted rather irresponsibly and did not call me or even brief *Dr. PN D* about when I am coming. I reached there and had expected someone to be there at the station. There was no help in the new city. My initial reaction was disbelief, followed by anger and concern. Now the problem is how to track them down? In those days we had no cell phones and I had no idea whom to contact.

I used my brain and did not panic. When things get tough the tough get going. I was able to locate the team, using logic. It wa late at night and I was tired. I took a room in a hotel. Next day I went to the state legislative assembly. In those days the security was less and I was easily able to go inside. I had no name or any contact person to reach out to, just made a few inquiries with the security and was able to reach the right person. By this time and stroke of luck, *Dr PN D* and RR(S) came to see this guy. They came in the university bus and we all connected

This year again we were better prepared and had more clarity. We easily won the zonal championship and reached the national final. In the finals hosted in Delhi, we were runners up, won the silver medal. It was certainly a much better performance but still short of the ultimate gold.

In the second year we had allowed the sort of turncoat college team which ditched us to rejoin. So the number of participants per college dropped to 6. Since *Dr. PN D* was there, I think we were in a position of advantage and got a chance to have one more candidate from our college. This new participant was *Red S A*. At that time I knew him just as a junior in our college and later we became friends.

As we moved into 3rd year. A lot of the senior team members graduated out and they started playing games. I had hoped they would support or atleast stay neutral but they had other thoughts and turned hostile. I don't know why but they may be having a feeling that this belonged to them and the team could not be sent or the tournament held without them. They acted unfairly. Instead of acting as a coach or mentor they tried to sabotage the preparation.

I am not sure who all was involved but someone was clearly helping another University to act as a competitor and giving all our valuable trade secrets out. The cheapest thing they did was poison the minds of the girl students. There was a letter written to the university authorities signed by these girls saying they felt unsafe with the new team. This was like a bolt from the blue, totally unexpected and what surprised me was that so many of the girls signed this. I thought we had good relations with them and would not become party of a false propaganda and resist any stupid move. Unfortunately; I proved wrong and the herd mentality changed the whole scenario against us.

We had now got to do a lot more groundwork and some PR exercises. Wecertainly had some hiccups and a few issues did crop up. With help of Dr. P N D had to take the authorities into confidence. We acted smartly and managed to get a new balanced team together. Some girls who were doing propaganda against us dropped out but most of the veterans joined us back.

In the zonal competition a few days before we were to perform a new internal problem surfaced. One of the girl students was not happy with what was happening and had an ego issue. She unexpectedly stood up and created a ruckus in the team rehearsal. She was not being singled out or sidelined.. In the middle of the training she stood up and angrily decided to boycott the proceedings. She announced names of 2 more friends who would boycott. We decided to discipline her and throw her out of any role she was to play. Her friends did not support this drama.

Third year we had learnt a lot and thus improved our performance but due to external political issues we were the zonal runners up and failed to qualify for the finals. There were clearly very controversial and security related national level topics touched. Which was a clear and blatant violation of the rules of conduct. So we gave a written complaint which was upheld and that year the finals were cancelled.

Overall, the competition was fun. we got a chance to see so many new places, experience some new adventures and helped me and many teammates to get University Colour and even the University Roll of Honour. I would certainly like to say our sincere team effort and hard work gave us new status in the Inter-University tournament. We got a lot more recognition and respect. We formed a new bond of friendship and a kind of loose group as we all enjoyed each other's company and had something in common to talk about.

TEN

# The Cricket Match

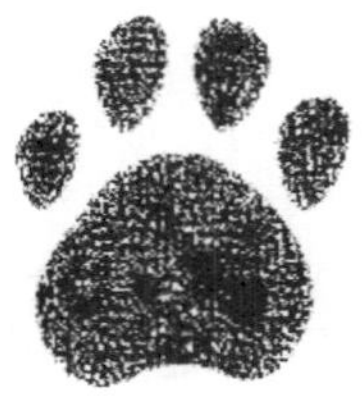

In our youthful University days, we all like to have fun. We love to entertain and play. Out of all the games played in India cricket is one of the most popular. Cricket gained a lot of popularity especially after India won the 1983 world cup, later also got the chance to host the 1987 cup. It was like a cricket fever in the country's youth. The match I am talking about happened soon after the world cup. The atmosphere was charged and the players were being appreciated and made to look like demigods.

Almost every student all over the country starts taking the game seriously. The thinking that he/ she is an undiscovered talent. Soon he/ she will be spotted. Media adds fuel to it and comes with attractive stories of some players rising from the street to play for the national side. Our university and its students were no exception. We all began to see ourselves as the next Kapil Dev, Sunil Gavaskar.

Lot more tournaments are held With this background an intra college tournament is organised. As far as I remember never before and never after did any such event take place. Either, there was no initiative or the authorities simply refused to approve it. This series was announced out of blue and we were all excited to participate. It was truly a great WOW! moment.

I was also thrilled as it would give me a chance to ape my cricket heroes. There would be a chance to use the whole kit - gloves, pad, guard and I would play on a professionally prepared cricket pitch. We used to play a lot in the park, and streets but never on the ground with the full cricket kit. I could not stop feeling happy. I would play for my class. In the past, in my school I had attempted to play for my class but unfortunately, I did badly. I was out on the very first ball.

I would like to mention as a side note here, that in street cricket, my brother was a good fast bowler. We would face his speed without the kit, especially no pads or gloves and this affected the batting technique. We became more careful of our legs and hands. The leather ball comes fast, it hits and hurts so in a situation like this you were forced to play in a way to protect your legs and hands. I developed some bad batting style that I could not get rid of. knew something needed to be improved but I did not know what and how. I saw some cricket matches to see what could be done but had no coach. I was inspired by great players like Bedi. I worked on becoming a spin bowler.

In this college game my buddy *Raj S* was selected as the class team captain. He wasn the obvious and appropriate choice. He had a good background and had represented our university. I believe he was the only player from our class who had the honour. I was happy for him and expected I would get extra importance in the team. My buddy was calling the shots and making all the decisions. Later as we will see my hopes were badly dashed.

We were playing against the team which was our one-year juniors. They also boosted some good players in it. One of the players, Jaty *S* had also donned the university role. He had represented the university team and had a good reputation. He was a good player and particularly a good bowler. Overall both the opposing team looked strong. We were playing for fun and it was less of a competition. Who really cares for the results even if you lose or win.

Before this match, we got an opportunity to practise in the Univ. nets. These nets had many more players apart from us. We had a chance to rub shoulders with these local stars. The interaction with them was short and lasted only for a few days. Some new skills were honed. I remember I faced a good spin bowler and I thought I could hit him out of the stadium. Only to balloon the ball in the air and make an easy catch. I used this god given time to learn the ball movement of the seam and in the air.

In my street, I used to ball well and was never taken lightly. I was looking to become better. I was a reasonably good batsman. I loved to play more on the leg side to the point I used to cross bat. This bad habit I had picked up protecting my legs. I was also an agile fielder. Overall I was a good player for this level of the game.

While preparing in the nets, I could feel I was out of form and lacked the soft touch. I needed more practice and some coaching but that was not an option. We lacked the luxury of time and resources. We were only here for an inter class game and not for anything big.

On the scheduled day, I remember very clearly the weather was good. It was a wonderful sunshine and a very pleasant day. The temperature was quite ambient, not too warm or cold. I don't remember which month it was but the time was certainly a bright early to mid-afternoon. The venue of the match was played at the main sports complex. There were two pitches almost side to side. Considering the low importance attached to this game we were not allowed to use the main pitch. It was always well maintained and usually kept reserved for the bigger tournaments.

 It was decided to have a 25 over match, this would end the game early. I don't remember how much was the target. They batted well and we had fun bowling to the opponents. I absolutely would have loved to be given an opportunity to bowl. Unfortunately, I looked on and waited when my time would come. The captain would hand me the desirable red leather ball. I waited and watched all the20 overs as long as the other team was on the crease. I was not given a chance to throw the ball over. I saw the wickets tumble runs being made but I was totally ignored.

Remember, all this happened when *Raj S* was at the helm of affairs. He was my close friend and in the past, we had played together. He had seen me perform well as a baller. It was baffling and it is still not clear why he did not call me? Not even once. I can only guess maybe he did not have faith and did not trust my skills. At times in the game especially when they were going strong, he looked confused and struggling for options. Whom to give the next chance. It never came to me. I should have asked him before or during the match. I didn't do it, I was stuck between my ego and giving my friend a free hand. I should acknowledge I felt hurt and did not like his attitude. I kept quiet and did not point it out, or protest.

I would admit that I felt my abilities were overlooked by my friend. I have a victim mentality where I want to feel poor me. I started feeling maybe I lacked the skills. How I have been ignored at other such things. I remember he asked one boy, Venkat, to come forward. Venkat 5 pitched wide balls in an over of 6. Later, he proudly boasted he is a fantastic bowler and only gave away 4 runs. You count the total damage 5 extra runs, 4 runs and 4 extra balls. If I remember all these happenings even decades later it is certain it has and continues to create a significant impact on my mind.

Being in the playing 11 guarantees you a chance to bat. I don't remember at which number I batted but it was certainly towards the middle order. How many runs I actually scored that day faded in memory. I certainly did not get a duck. As I stepped on to bat, I was facing *Jay,* a good reputed bowler. Captain of the opponents. I came to bat with full gear, pads and gloves. minus the helmet which was considered a luxury.

As I came to the pitch before I took my guard. I loudly made funny jokes or humorous gibes, "don't you dare get me out you MFs".. As we all knew the game was less competitive and more fun. I do recall all the details only bits and pieces. In some parts I do recollect the first ball I could not read and I came down the pitch to hit the ball. I missed the ball, missed the wicket and the keeper's gloves. I had fun, scored a few runs hitting the ball all over and I think I did get out.

As far as my memory goes we lost the match. I don't remember our or their total team totals or the individual scores or even the wickets taken by players. What is still in my mind is that it was a narrow defeat. Being a round-robin we were knocked out Later the junior team progressed and played with the seniors and won the second time. They ended up being the college champions.

A couple of side notes I was so out of touch with the game that I could not do a good fielding. I was always proud of my agility and ability to take good sharp catches, block the ball on the ground. I had expected I would do well. That day I was slow and sluggish and did a lousy job of stopping runs. The Vice Captain *Mon D* was not happy; he advised me that I should throw my body into the ball. I must have done a sloppy job to get noticed and the advice. My performance cost the team valuable runs. I did try but in a game or anything else in life things just don't happen in a flash. I used to be inspired watching fielders like Azar. To field well you need to practise hard and only then do you perform well.

This match took place about 30 years ago. Some of the incidents which create an impact good or bad are fresh like yesterday. It certainly means something must have touched my soul. I still feel *RS* did not honour my skills, it showed up as a lack of faith in my ability to ball. On days we had student strikes we would go and play cricket. On more than one occasion he had joined us.

As a mature human being, I need to overcome this hurt and I don't think I will or should talk to him now. It is too late and will do anyone any good, we continued to be friends and are still close.

# End

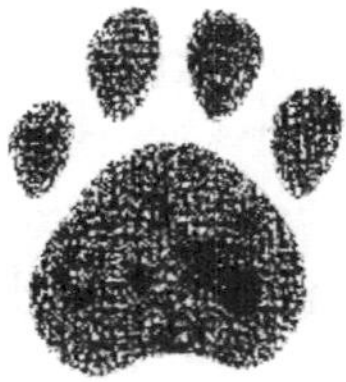

As I complete my first public book, I am feeling extremely excited and very happy. For me, it is a big mission that has been accomplished. I have one more thing knocked off my to-do list. I have written before but they were more professional essays and mostly on scientific topics. I always wanted to write something simple like stories, and light reading. Make some new friends. It will be very appropriate to sincerely thank Geetika and Beeja education for helping me come this far.

In this book, I have tried to use simple incidents to define complex questions in life. The wise and enlightened have always stated that life is just a series of simple occurrences bundled together in one common chord- time. In this book, I tried to share some of these occurrences and have fun.

I hope the reader can connect with the theme and enjoy this journey with me. This book and series which I plan to write in the future will illustrate a well known simple concept: you plant a seed and it will mature into a tree tomorrow. My inception happened in 1987 and then in face of all adverse internal and external factors grew to have a decent and successful career.

Things in life always begin this way, one innocent step at a time. I would compare this with an onion. You peel it year by year and sometimes it even makes you cry. When the job of peeling and cutting is done, we are privileged to enjoy the taste of the food. Life is a bouquet of flavours and emotions, which bring both pain and pleasure.

In my book, I have shown some of the major challenges I faced and how I overcame and triumphed. This happened to me repeatedly when things looked bleak and circumstances were not in my favour, somebody unexpectedly jumped in as a saviour. This help and guidance mostly saved the day. Then, it is not true that every time I had a messiah and I was successful. We had our set of failures originating. They originated from poor judgement. Maybe if I was smarter, more courageous, planned things and had the guts to say no, we would have had different results.

This book is mainly about student days. When I was young things were very romantic and beautiful. At that age and with a heart full of love it is very natural there is an affair. I believe most students experience this attraction. Many of these relationships are temporary and may not last. However, some of these encounters and friendships could leave a good taste and be a cherished memory.

In this book, I have tried to write about the importance of feelings and emotions and how they define our destiny. Incidents happen and situations arise. Our reactions to the occasion rather than the incidents themselves are more important. This response will be unique to an individual and he/ she will arrive at a conclusion.

This conclusion and subsequent action make a habit and a character. Which ultimately determines a destiny.

I have begun to enjoy writing. There are a lot more to write and many more incidents which I would like to share. Due to the paucity of space and time, we have to end here.

I promise I will continue my efforts and come back with a sequel. Many more interesting stories to follow.

# About the Author

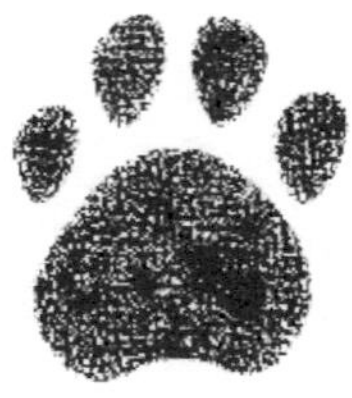

I am Pushproop Brar, a practising Veterinarian and have been proudly serving livestock for nearly 30 years. I am a graduate of PAU, Ludhiana. I am currently living and helping the animals in Canada.

I have a lot of love and affection for animals. I shall continue to serve this important sector in the foreseeable future. When I joined the profession, I had a vision and have always worked toward those who are considered meek. I am fulfilling my moral and ethical role in society.

I always feel satisfied that my efforts have gone towards the values, I truly believe in and stand by. I have been lucky to be in different areas of veterinary medicine, been a clinician, in private practice and as a regulator served in different government roles.

During this time, I have had many experiences and I would say have a lot of volunteer learning opportunities. This has made me more mature and wiser.

My plan is to help in uplifting the profession. I always educate people about how to understand our furry friends and take care of the animals. We cohabit the biosphere, so smooth and cooperative living is mandatory.

I have a wonderful family and I am married to a beautiful lady and proud father of two awesome kids.